Acupuncture Blueprint for Success

Transform Your Practice Growth 10x and Clinical Results 10x with Structural Alignment Acupuncture

Regan Archibald Lac, CSSAc
Functional Medicine Practitioner

Acupuncture Blueprint for Success

Printed by:
90-Minute Books
302 Martinique Drive
Winter Haven, FL 33884
www.90minutebooks.com

Published in the United States of America

Book ID: 161106-00601

ISBN-13: 978-1945733550
ISBN-10: 1945733551

This book is a dedication to all of my mentors who have steered me into a more fulfilling and abundant future than I could have ever imagined.

Here's What's Inside...

Introduction

According to research, 1.5 billion people on the planet suffer from some kind of chronic pain, including 11% of the American population. The Seattle based rapper, Macklemore, released an emotionally engaging song about the abuse of the pharmaceutical companies and the addictions that so many of us lose our lives to. The hook done by Ariana DeBoo goes, "My drug dealer was a doctor, doctor, had the plug from Big Pharma, Pharma. He said he would heal me, heal me, but he only gave me problems, problems." The solution to pain has been to swallow another pill that has been advertised as "non-addictive"—think Purdue Pharma with OxyContin.

From 1999 to 2010, pain prescriptions quadrupled and it's still on a steady rise. You and I have seen the grey faces that walk into our offices desperately wanting to kick the habit. They walk in our offices dismantled of power by their addiction, the shallow look in their eyes, their quavering voices, the hands that tremble, lost relationships—all from their addiction. The worst thing about this growing pain epidemic is that people like you and I have solutions that can stop the problem before it festers into a life ending pill binge.

Another study released in 2015 by the *Lancet*, found that "95% of the world's population has health problems and 1/3 of those have more than five chronic conditions." I wish I had all of the answers to the worldwide health problems, but the use of pharmaceuticals and invasive surgery has run its course. There are more people than ever who need your help, and now is the time to offer a fresh new approach. If you are reading this, then you are part of the solution and my job is to help reveal some ways you can amplify your results with your patients. Now more than ever before, you can make a bigger impact for the 95% of people who suffer. You can't confront the problem without getting an entirely new set of capabilities. To get the results that are necessary, we need to think differently about the way we've been practicing and running our clinics.

In *Acupuncture Blueprint for Success*, I'm going to share with you why the vast majority of acupuncturists struggle to get their practices launched and how you can avoid that trap. I will share with you how I have been able to overcome my own struggles of trying to build a successful acupuncture practice and what I learned along the way that has allowed me to grow one of the most game-changing, innovative practices in the country called East West Health.

I will also share how you can use a brand new treatment technique, called Structural Alignment Acupuncture in your practice and how you will be able to stand out as the expert in multiple areas. For you to succeed, you need to master both acupuncture and becoming an entrepreneur because you can't have one without the other in today's economic environment.

Enjoy the book!

The purpose of my writing this book is to open a door of opportunity to you that you may not know exists when it comes to growing a viable acupuncture practice, and that helps more people than you could ever imagine. Healthcare in America is broken; it's you and I who hold the answers for creating new horizons for individuals looking for better answers to their conditions.

You are the answer to this massive problem but probably are unaware that you can make ten times the impact that you are now with some of the principles taught in this book.

This book is not meant to be an exhaustive text on Structural Alignment Acupuncture, nor will it provide all the tools necessary to grow a transformative acupuncture practice, but it will give you the ability to take the first step towards a bolder future.

To Your Success!

Regan Archibald, Lac, CSSAc

Your Present and Future Purpose

To prepare yourself mentally to transform your practice and your life, keep your journal handy so you can write down new ideas which come to you while you study this material. Become 100% committed to taking action on the new things you are learning. Some concepts will come naturally, and others may take some further thought before they sink in. If you feel stuck, don't hesitate to email me at **regan@gowellness.com**, or come to one of my live training sessions so you can learn first-hand. Reading this material will only get you so far, come learn in a hands-on way.

I would like to share the eight key mindsets that will allow you to grow faster. When you can apply these mindsets to your own practice, they will allow you the freedom to innovate and try new things. The eight mindsets I have discovered will transform your acupuncture practice are as follows:

Mindset #1: Your purpose is to help as many people as possible get as healthy as possible with natural medicine. Every day, you are making advancements in your ability to grow as a practitioner and entrepreneur to create healthcare that will make a bigger impact.

Mindset #2: You are committed to taking 100% responsibility for your own health and well-being. You wake up every day with a renewed commitment to experiment on yourself so that you can discover where real health can be found.

Mindset #3: Your target is to find and treat the root cause because you realize that treating symptoms will only get you so far. Your examination, testing, lab reviews, and learning are always expanding and you are using the best resources possible to identify and remove causal agents.

Mindset #4: You enter every patient encounter in a heart-centered flow state which allows you to be creative and to deeply connect with those you serve. Your work brings you significant enjoyment and you feel refreshed by your ability to provide meaningful care.

Mindset #5: You see that having certainty and clear communication creates 90% of your results. What you say is powerful and can transform an ordinary treatment into a life changing experience because of the confidence you inspire your patients with.

Mindset #6: You see that office systems continually lead to better outcomes because they provide a container which allows you to perform your best work.

Systems create a more meaningful patient experience and reduce your workload.

Mindset #7: You understand that healing is a unique process every individual must go through in order to grow. You are simply there as a guide who can direct the patient on the correct path for lasting results that move them in a brighter, healthier future.

Mindset #8: You are finding breakthroughs in new and expanding technology which includes new acupuncture methods, communication tools, office systems and diagnostic testing. You can see the freedom that technology can provide you and your patients when it is properly utilized.

These eight mindsets will keep your purpose, intention and impact firmly rooted in what your goals are. They will also remind you to take new actions when you become trapped in your current ways of doing things. In the future, discover your own mindsets that have created more meaning and freedom in your life and write them down and live by them.

Learning Seitai Shinpo Acupuncture

When I moved to Hawaii to study acupuncture and Chinese medicine, I would often have people ask me where I was from and what brought me to the island.

I would explain that the reason I was on the island was to learn how to practice holistic medicine and acupuncture. Ninety percent of the time, a huge smile would come across their faces and they would talk about their experience with Dr. Chieko Maekawa. Wherever I went, people would talk about her and how they'd seen miraculous changes. After the third or fourth time hearing about her, I realized I had to meet this healer.

My first attempts to introduce myself and become a student of hers were shut down. She wasn't taking any students and didn't need any help at her clinic. I was finally able to get the president of my school involved, and so doors were opened for me and some of my classmates to attend an elective course taught at her clinic. Our job was to clean the clinic and take notes from her fascinating lectures. A short time later, Dr. Maekawa could see my sincere desire to learn and invited me to shadow her while she treated patients. I was instructed to, "not move the air" and to be a "fly on the wall" so that I didn't distract from what she was doing.

I apprenticed with Dr. Maekawa for more than three years and saw miraculous recoveries from some of the most difficult conditions imaginable.

I also was able to learn a unique form of structural alignment acupuncture called Seitai Shinpo, which translates as correct posture acupuncture method.

Seeing Dr. Maekawa practice Seitai Shinpo opened my eyes to this entirely new process of looking at acupuncture. Now if you're like me and you enjoy sports medicine, enjoy orthopedics, and like to understand the mechanics of the body, then this system of acupuncture will resonate with you.

This technique will allow you to simply use needles to realign the spine and reverse autoimmune conditions. I'd like to give you some of the history of this treatment and how it was invented.

My lineage starts with Sawada Ken and goes to Keizo Hashimoto, who was a medical doctor, 1897–1993. Sawada Ken lived 1877–1938. And then Daiichi Sorimachi, who is still practicing in Tokyo. He's approaching 80. And then my teacher, Dr. Chieko Maekawa, who is over 80! And then I was the very first American acupuncturist certified in Seitai Shinpo acupuncture. I'm one of the founding members of the Seitai Shinpo Acupuncture Foundation.

Now, Structural Alignment Acupuncture is a little different than Seitai Shinpo Acupuncture as you'll learn. In my 12 years of practice, I have modified this system of acupuncture so that I could help more people than I could by sticking to traditional Seitai Shinpo, which requires 45 minutes to an hour of time in the room with each patient. In making this shift, I was able to open up my schedule so I could treat up to eight patients every hour and still maintain phenomenal results.

Getting Your Practice Off the Ground

In my Acupuncture Blueprint for Success training module, I will be teaching you many of the successful actions which have allowed me to create seven-figure practices, several times over. I've helped multiple practitioners do this. A lot of you know me from my Lotus events. I've done trainings on Structural Alignment Acupuncture. I've done trainings on Detoxification and Weight Loss and on Hormones and Four Body Types. Trainings on Reversing Autoimmune Conditions, Supporting Genetics, Correcting Heart Disease, and Thyroid conditions. I also have created treatments that influence the body's own stem cells with acupuncture and Chinese herbs to enhance the healing response.

I deliver impactful functional medicine trainings throughout the year with Go Wellness, and I spend my spare time developing content for my Healthcare Entrepreneur program which teaches natural healthcare providers how to be entrepreneurs. I currently have four clinics throughout Utah and have one of the most incredible teams on the planet! This book will focus on you as an acupuncturist, and I hope to be able to meet you in the future.

Once you're able to help forty, fifty, sixty, maybe even a hundred patients a week, then we can start adding in other service centers and then you can start bringing in associates to perform acupuncture for you. You can start bringing in other key players for marketing, for managing your books. You can bring in a Health Coach and we've got a whole training on that.

There are so many different avenues down which you can take your practice, once you've got this key component complete: get a strong acupuncture base, help them get better faster, then they will start talking about you and your success will soar. I found this out early on in my practice. In 2017, this is easier than it's ever been with all of the free outlets with social media which allow your patients to easily tell their friends about your clinic through a simple review or post.

Introduction of the Acupuncture Genius and Legend

I learned Seitai Shinpo Acupuncture, and I found it to be enlightening beyond anything I'd ever experienced in acupuncture because of the experience I had with the treatment.

In this treatment, your left hand, your guided hand, is always on the patient. So you're always palpating. You're feeling for indurations, which is an "increase in the fibrous elements in tissue commonly associated with inflammation and marked by loss of elasticity and pliability ... sclerosis ... a hardened mass or formation." These indurations, when detected early enough, will feel like a sesame seed in the sub-dermal layer—this is your target. The more indurations you can resolve, the greater the results. You will find that acupuncture points haven't always been fixed on the body the way we learned them in school, so fine-tuning your palpation is the best way to locate the right point.

You also find indurations to understand what muscles are causing that spinal misalignment; then you needle the areas of contractions so the patient's body comes back to center. Once their physical body is centered, their emotional and spiritual alignment will also center.

This is one of the deepest aspects of Structural Alignment Acupuncture: to allow the patient and the practitioner to become centered and present together.

The path to diagnose the four patterns of contraction starts with looking at the superior ridge of the iliac crest. If your right hip is contracted and your right shoulder is contracted, that's going to put pressure on your liver. If your left shoulder's down and your left hip's raised up, that's going to cause constipation. It's also going to cause heart issues. And if your chest is contracted inward, then your lungs are affected and that's going to put a burden on your cardiovascular system. We will be diving deeper into these patterns throughout the book.

If you can start looking at Structure Alignment, there are some very cool things you can do with it. And it's going to enhance your patients' confidence in you.

Patients ask me, "Do you think I should go to a chiropractor?" once I have examined the patterns of misalignment along their spine. I usually say, "You know, it's fine. They do great work, but I can realign your spine with my needle." This is the essence of what Structural Alignment Acupuncture will do, but it's in a very comfortable way.

It's one of the most comfortable acupuncture treatment methods you'll ever experience.

Everyone who I've administered this treatment to says nothing but how good they feel. They feel centered. They feel grounded.

So, it's all about connecting the brain, the heart, and the kidneys—all of the systems in your body—and that's what Structural Alignment Acupuncture is designed around.

My teacher, Dr. Chieko Maekawa, always teases that she stole this information from Daiichi Sorimachi. He's been published in the *Northern Journal of Japanese Acupuncture*. I too have a couple of published articles in there on this method as well. What Dr. Maekawa found is that my teacher, Daiichi Sorimachi, my grandmaster, he would not write down the points. So my teacher was very scrupulous in ascertaining which points he's using most frequently to realign the spine.

Now, one thing that Daiichi Sorimachi was trained in was Sotai-ho. For those of you who are familiar with Keizo Hashimoto, he's the inventor of Sotai-ho. He was a medical doctor in Japan and he realized that the pharmaceutical drugs he was offering his patients were not getting them better. He noticed that the traditional healers, the practitioners of Shiatsu, of Moxibustion, of

Acupuncture, and herbal medicine, were actually getting better results than he was.

What he sought out to do was to create his own methodology of healing and so Keizo Hashimoto created what's called the Sotai-ho Movement Therapy.

Now, Sotai-ho is when you are moving your body in the path of least resistance. So, for example, if I pulled my right hamstring. Then with Sotai-ho, I would practice moving my left hamstring and stretching it rather than stretching on the side that got injured. So, it's completely opposite of, for example, physical therapy. The other movement you'll do is stretching to the left and then you stretch to the right like you're a cat. Which way feels better? And then you stretch to the side that feels the best. It's sort of interesting. It's like water. It's the wu wei Principle.

You know, follow the flow. Follow the path. And that's what Sotai-ho is built around. It's built around four principles, which are proper thinking, proper movement, proper eating, and proper breathing. Dr. Hashimoto advocated specific stretches and exercises at night before bed where he'd do abdominal massage and deep breathing. He also advocated more of a macrobiotic based diet. But, Sotai-ho was what my grandmaster, Daiichi Sorimachi, was initially inspired by. Daiichi Sorimachi combined the Sawada Ken style of Acupuncture with Sotai-ho.

Sawada Ken, his whole philosophy was focused around treating points on the back shu, primarily with Moxibustion. For Daiichi Sorimachi, those are the points he utilized with his patients for years. These points along the bladder channel are very profound in enhancing spinal alignment. When my teacher, Dr. Maekawa, saw Dr. Sorimachi using these points, she was inspired. She decided to make him write something down. So the very first thing he talked about was the possible pattern of contraction in the body. That's one of the first tools we train you on in our hands-on course, how to diagnose those patterns of contraction.

Before you administer the SAA, use key opening points so the energy has a direction to flow into. You can use moxa on San Jiao 4 on the right side and Ren 12. Then anchor the energy into the legs with stomach 36 or gallbladder 34. The needle and moxa large intestine 10 or 11. These were some of the main points that Sawada Ken used for years, and Sawada Ken was famous for treating patients with very chronic conditions— patients on their deathbed, reviving them. Also, he was very famous for bridging the gap between Western medicine and Acupuncture.

The traditional medicines in Japan in the early 1900s, late 1800s, were starting to be frowned upon as there was more of a Western influence coming in.

The main points Sawada Ken would use were urinary bladder 20, 23, 25, 27 and he'd use urinary bladder 32 for any reproductive issues. In the upper back points, he would use urinary bladder 18, 17, 16, 15. Urinary bladder 44, San Jiao 15, Gallbladder 20, Bladder 10, Du 20. Those are all points that he found to be very effective for reversing autoimmunity problems.

I had the privilege and honor of spending about two months showing Dr. Maekawa that I was sincere in my efforts to learn from her. I wanted to train with her and I had a deep desire to be a devoted student. When she finally let me into her clinic, I was able to learn and apprentice under her for several years and I've been practicing this model and studying this system of Acupuncture for more than 15 years now.

What I found is that you will get better results with a quicker response in less time than if you used TCM acupuncture, meridian therapy, Master Tung or distal needling.

During my internship and resident work in Hawaii, I researched the results of several types of acupuncture and was steadfast in learning which system worked the best. I discovered that Sietai Shinpo would yield the best results overall.

Using this method of acupuncture, I was able to fill up my schedule with 40–50 patient visits per week in the first three months that I began my practice. I then developed tools which allowed me to see over 200 patients per week while maintaining very consistent results. I would love to show you how you can do the same.

Let's Chat, How to Get in Touch with Regan

Fast forward to the present day. I'm the founder of East West Health. I've created four incredible clinics in Utah. I'm also the founder of the educational platform and healthcare entrepreneur training program called Go Wellness. We run seminars all over the country, from L.A. to Brooklyn to Salt Lake City, Utah. I've got three amazing kids. An incredible wife who teaches me more about life, business and organization than any paid coach has. We have a really cool dog named Andre. I own lots of mountain bikes and I love snowboarding. I live in Park City, Utah and I'd love to meet you face to face.

We've got amazing things to offer. My goal in creating this book is to help inspire the acupuncture community into looking at a new way of treating the body with spinal alignment. I think it's a brilliant method. It's genius. And I want to get the word out there.

I'm so happy you're reading this and I hope that in the few words I have shared that you are finding new inspiration to practice your craft in a new way. If this is something that you feel like you want to dig in deeper with, then email me at regan@gowellness.com, and let's change the world together.
I help practitioners create transformative clinics which are incredibly profitable and are fun to practice in.

I also train at live events as well. You'll find our calendar at gowellness.com. You can also go to acupunctureblueprint.com and you'll get all the details about this specific course. I've personally created several training courses which can motivate and inspire you to create more value for your patients with programs that help you succeed at levels you never thought you could reach. These programs will help you implement Structural Alignment Acupuncture, functional medicine, and stem cell therapy into your practice. They will help you learn how to build a business that's going to last long after you're gone.

My purpose is to change the landscape of healthcare in America, because too many people are on drugs unnecessarily and too many people are getting costly surgeries. I think we need to change that message, and you're the ones to do it.

I'm honored you have read this far.

Bridging Ancient Wisdom with New Methodology

Your 2500-Year-Old Secret to Successful Acupuncture Outcomes

This chapter is focused on diagnostics and patient communication. It's going to help propel you to the next level in your practice because as you gain more confidence in your diagnosis and learn how to communicate your findings, you will have a deeper influence with your patients. Let's first dive into the *Yellow Emperor's Classic*. This book was written over two thousand years ago, so it's not a new release. This is a conversation; it's a very poetic book.

I know many of you have read it and studied it in school. This is where Qi Bo is talking to the Yellow Emperor Huang Di, and what he's saying is, "What is the key to acupuncture?" That's what Huang Di was looking for is, some insights on why it's so important, why it's so valuable, and how it works, because acupuncture, historically, wasn't used as extensively as it is today in Traditional Chinese Medicine.

What Qi Bo responded with was, "The key to acupuncture is, first of all, concentrate and focus. You must perceive the deficiencies and accesses of the organs, and the nine pulses, then you can administer acupuncture."

Now this is just as true today as it was back then. In fact, today I think we have more distractions than I'm sure Qi Bo had. I'm sure he didn't have a smartphone pinging him every three minutes and that meditation and finding a quiet spot was a little easier for him than it may be for us. What's true is that when you focus and when you concentrate, what you do is slow down time. This is exactly how I am able to treat hundreds of patients in a short amount of time.

When you are present and fully connected with your patients, what they experience is something that's transcendent, because once again, you're not just looking for a result of, "Let's get rid of your pain as quickly as possible," although that helps. What we're really trying to do, we're stepping into the area where we are providing a transformative experience for our patients. We are correcting underlying imbalances.

The only way you can do that is when you're a 100% present with them. I find that you can't be present if you're not focused, and if you're not clear on what you're looking to accomplish in your treatments, then you won't get the results you could have. No matter what style of acupuncture you practice, your focus and concentration matters just as much now as it did 2500 years ago.

With the structure alignment acupuncture method, one of the best things I found about it is it has always allowed me to concentrate and focus, because I'm not worried so much about the patterns and the syndrome, and am I using a Jing Well Point, or is this a Yuan Source Point, or do I need to focus on the Lung Meridian, or the Kidneys, which is it? What I find is, I can just really dive in and get down to the heart of the issue with my patients, because I'm simply letting my fingers guide the treatment.

Now I'm looking for indurations in their spine, I've checked for distortions, I've done orthopedic tests, so I have a very good understanding of where the misalignments are in their spine. Then I'm using my intuition, and I'm using my words as if they were acupuncture needles, because as many of you know, your communication is more powerful than a needle.

Those words have very succinct powerful meaning behind them if you're concentrating and focusing. If you're distracted, if you're thinking about your date tonight, or you're thinking about the fight you had with your lady or your man, that's not going to help lend itself to your intention and your words. Words have powerful vibrations and carry context for everything you are doing.

In structure alignment acupuncture, you confidently walk into the room fully prepared and fully aware of what's going on with that patient's body. You're using your hand to palpate along the spine, and you're keeping that hand on the person's body the entire time. You breathe with them and peer deep into their soul. This process will become very intuitive and natural because right inside of your body are all the tools you need to be incredibly psychic in very little time.

As you release those Indurations, their spine starts to unlock from the bottom up. If you've studied Ayurvedic medicine, you know your root chakra is right around Bladder 32 and Ren 4. Once you open up that energy center, that lower Dantian, that's where the person starts to experience what it feels like to be a self-actualized human.

We're looking for transcendence, not only from a physical perspective but also an energetic and psychological perspective. Each needle, as it goes in, you're placing the needle very carefully. In fact, you're going right down to the transverse process on each vertebrae and needling deep into these points. The needle should be perpendicular and you will feel a gummy sensation that tugs on the needle when you've reached the proper depth.

This technique is not taught in schools and is very satisfying to your patient. It feels like a deep itch has been scratched and the amount of pain relief is substantial.

Now remember, those points are one cun above the traditional Chinese acupuncture point. Make sure you're getting the training in. In our online training course, you'd learn all this, but it's best to do hands-on during our live sessions.

As you're experiencing these moments with your patients, you have no question in your mind that by using Structural Alignment Acupuncture, you're going to get light years ahead of where you are now, because you have points that can literally transform a person who's got autoimmune diseases like Graves and Hashimoto's.

One of my patients recently called us and said, "You won't believe it Regan, my Endocrinologist just ran my labs, and my thyroid numbers, my (TPO) thyroid peroxidase antibodies registered at zero. I have no immune reaction. I am in remission, he's never seen this.

We have these types of turnarounds often, and along with acupuncture, we're working on lifestyle, nutrition, but we're also using the spine, and especially the cervical spine in thyroid issues.

Diagnosing the 4 Patterns of Contraction

When you're going into the room with a patient, the first thing you want to do is to put your hands on the Upper Iliac Spine. You want to just see, "Okay, which side is contracted most ... Which hipbone is higher than the other one?" Once you can see that, you will say to your patients, "Wow, that right hip is really higher than the left," then that's the side that you want to needle a little more aggressively. Pull out about an inch and a half needle, maybe a 36 gauge, is typically what I'll use. When you get more Jedi with this, I use a three-inch needle, typically. And then you will needle each of the points along the Bladder channel that you find indurations in, but stay focused on the primary points.

You're going to palpate around the lumbar spine to find the Large Intestine Shu. That will be one up from there. You're going to draw a line, the top of the Iliac Crest, a straight line across. You're going to find the most contracted side. The space between the spinous process, typically between about L2 and L3, and you're going to needle that bladder point, and you're going to go straight in, all the way in. Inch and a half to three inches, depending on your skill level, and your comfort level, and you're going to go nice and slow. Very, very easy. You're not forcing things, you're not thrusting the needle.

You're not breaking the tissue up, you're going very, very thin. Then you're going to go on the Small Intestine Shu and then Bladder 32, followed by the Kidney Shu and then Spleen Shu to complete the lower back points.

Every needle insertion is just a nice, subtle entry. You're going to feel the release in the form of a muscle twitch in a lot of cases. You will also feel the patient relax and stop resisting the needle insertion. You're going to feel an energetic buzz on that needle, and then you're going to go to the next point. Maybe you'll do the point on the left side, then one on the right. Just balance your needling so you don't move their spine too quickly. Start by needling the contracted side of the Large Intestine Shu, then you're going to move down two Cun, and you're going to find the Small Intestine Shu.

This is the most important point for realigning the entire spine, the Small Intestine Shu. Typically, that can be found by palpating just medial to the spinous process of the PSIS; Posterior Superior Iliac Spine.

Once you get into that groove, it's the SI joint, you'll needle directly perpendicular and you'll feel a gummy sensation when the needle hits the spot, and that gumminess is what we're aiming for. You're going to be palpating the point. You're going to be feeling for those little indurations.

An induration feels like a little sesame seed under your finger. You're going to needle this area 1–3" perpendicularly.

Now you've effectively needled those points, you're going to move to Bladder 32. Now, Bladder 32 is not always an easy point to find, especially if someone's big, and a lot of Americans are, but you're going to find that Second Foramen in the Sacrum. That second Sacral Foramen is going to unlock some magic, because Bladder 32 is not only powerful for releasing back pain and sciatica, this point's going to unlock their reproductive energy, and their sexual energy. A lot of people have suppressed sexual energy. Bladder 32 is going to also help open up their entire spine. The Large Intestine Shu, that's going to help with diseases like Colitis and I've seen it help Diverticulitis.

There was a local Gastro-Intestinal doctor who would refer all his patients to me because he saw the impact I had on one of his patients who had Diverticulitis and Colitis. I worked with this patient for four months and asked him to return to his GI doctor for a colonoscopy. This patient agreed because he had been symptom-free for nearly two months and his colonoscopy came out normal. No signs of Diverticulitis or Colitis. Never in his career had he seen anyone reverse Diverticulitis and Colitis that was as severe as this patient's case.

This GI doctor started sending all his patients to me, and then he finally went into research because he got tired of his practice.

All I was doing was needling the large intestine and small intestine shu points, making nutritional modifications, and administering herbal medicine. Where does healing start from anyways? It starts from the gut. If you don't have the right diversity in your microbiome, if you've got a yeast overgrowth, parasites, maybe you've got some Klebsiella, or even your patients with CDIF, who are not willing to do a fecal matter transplant. Then these points; the Large Intestine and Small Intestine Shu, can be part of the therapy to reverse those conditions.

I can't tell you how many people say, "Wow, I got off the table and I immediately had a bowel movement. I've been constipated for a week." This is because I needled the left side with greater intensity than the right side, as the left side is where your descending colon can get contracted. When you properly needle those points, you get their bowel movements regulated. Someone with loose stools, you make sure that that right side contraction gets released, and their stools normalize. There's something about getting better blood flow to those points of the body, because blood flow is what acupuncture is all about. Energy and blood flow.

If you look at it from a very physiological perspective, yes we're eliciting a nerve response, but more importantly, what's happening is your body's nervous system is responding. It is calling the immune system to work and the immune system sees that, "Wow, there's a foreign object in the body. Let's get the blood rushing down into the area."

What we're doing with structural alignment is, not only are we getting the blood moving to the area, we're eliciting an immune response, the nerves are getting disengaged and disarmed so that they can communicate more freely to your brain. But the biggest thing that we're after is releasing the indurations, that little sesame seed in the muscle that when needled properly, explodes the massed cells and creates a cascade of a healing response. Then your body goes into a massive pain relief very quickly.

What also happens with those spindle cells, is they're controlling the contraction and relaxation of that muscle group, so you can have an entire Quadratus Lumborum muscle, completely open up, that's been locked up for decades. Where chiropractors can't open it up, physical therapists can't open up. It opens up on its own, just by needling that point perfectly.

This is the beauty of structural alignment acupuncture. You can help so many people do so many things that you never dreamed of if you just learn how to find these three main shu points.

I want you to go practice those, send me an email, tell me how it went, **info@gowellness.com**.

Understanding How to Look Deeper

The last chapter covered the basic needling techniques, and that's how you want to guide yourself for all of the points along the spine. Now, this process takes some very deep intuition, but it also is very enlightening because, once you hit the right point, you'll know it and the patient will know it. I think all of us have experienced that as practitioners. One of the main things we're trying to reverse in our society is the incredible amount of issues in the gut and the autoimmunity, the leaky gut. I'm sure you've studied that but what I've found is if you can have the hips aligned, a person's digestive system will be ten times healthier. Especially if you've already corrected their diet, tested their biome, and resolved any pathogenic growth factors.

With Structural Alignment Acupuncture, you feel euphoric. Many of you have probably experienced this after you've had a good massage or a great acupuncture treatment, but this specific style of needling will open up all the systems in your body.

Your Posture is a Reflection of Your Health and Psychology

Let's talk a minute about moving the body and about the importance of that, because think about how you're sitting right now. Now, are you sitting with your body hunched over? Is your head pushed forward? Are you looking at a computer screen? Are you driving and you've got your gangster lean going on while listening to Jay-Z or Tupac?

As you look at your posture, there is something to be said about your health. You think of a person who walks with dignity, they walk upright, they walk straight, with eyes that are focused. That's somebody who you trust as a leader. Take President Obama's walk during his last days in office for example. He was almost done with his presidency and he walked with straight dignity, his posture was correct, he was not slouched. He showed good, positive energy Whenever I go shopping or if I'm at the store, I watch the way a person walks because you can tell a lot about their confidence levels, about how they feel about themselves, their life, their vision, if they are future-oriented or are they stuck in the past? Our posture is just a reflection of what we think about our self.

Think about someone who has their left shoulder hunched over and contracted. That's going to affect their heart, so they may have a difficult time expressing themselves. Their timing may be off, they may laugh at inappropriate times or they may show up late for events. They may also be disorganized because their heart is not open. They may have a hard time expressing their personality and they may try to just be like someone who they're not. That could be one of the indicators. Someone who's got a lot of grief, their shoulders are going to hunch over, they're going to collapse their lungs, they won't be inspired, they're going to feel unmotivated, they're going to have thyroid issues. They're going to be your patients who are very tough to deal with. They're going to crave carbs. You can put out a loaf of bread and they will steal it because they crave bread! They'll hide it under their shirt and run out of your office because that's one of the symptoms that will show up when they're looking for motivation in food.

Somebody who's got a right hip that's contracted up, right shoulder down, that's going to affect their liver, and so they may be irritable, they may be inflexible, they may be very difficult to deal with psychologically. What I've found is, as you start to watch the patterns in the structure, you'll start to see people with low-back pain who tend to hunch over, they've got either Hypokyphosis or Hyperkyphosis.

They may have some issues with really having a purpose in life. Their kidneys will be shut off, so they won't really have a clear path to what they're supposed to do and they might not have the wisdom that's necessary, so they may be afraid to take risks.

They're the government workers who stay in the same job forever. They're some of us, in our profession, the acupuncturists who, they don't try anything different, they just keep doing the same thing and they hope their practice will grow. They don't try new marketing avenues, they don't go speak, they think marketing is dirty, that's above them because they're afraid, they're afraid to put themselves out there. You're not writing that book, you're not delivering that webinar, you're not doing the things that you know that you need to and getting your message out, and so we really have to watch our own posture, our own structure, and look into our behaviors.

Moving into a New Purpose

The Japanese movement therapy, Sotai Ho, is all designed around correct movement, thinking, eating, and breathing and my teachers, Dr. Maekawa and Daiichi Sorimachi, have used this approach clinically in creating Seitai Shinpo. I have modified Seitai Shinpo and call it Structural Alignment Acupuncture, because I'm actually looking at aligning things on multiple levels. Energetically, I'm looking at aligning it from a behavioral perspective, a nutritional level, and then a functional medicine level. Each one of the points I talk about, you'll see me weave in functional medicine. I think this is very important because this is the medicine of the future. Pretty soon, our patients will be walking in and they'll have a cyborg chip implanted and their smartphone which will be giving us minute-by-minute updates, so we'll have a real-time data as far as what's going on their body, and if you don't know how to understand that data, then you're going to be left behind.

I think acupuncture and Chinese medicine will be at the forefront of medicine when it comes to treating chronic disease. Currently in America, 86% of health care spending is used to treat the symptoms of chronic disease with acute medicine. We are using amazing tools to treat the wrong conditions. Allopathic medicine and acute care are amazing but are only half of the story. If we're going to make a big change in health care in America, then using functional medicine, stem cell therapy, and Structural Alignment Acupuncture in your clinic is a good start.

The acupuncture world will start looking at Structural Alignment Acupuncture as another viable acupuncture method. Just like the Richard

Tan method, or TCM, or Master Tung. This technique is just one more arrow in your quiver. I'm not saying it's better than any of those, I'm saying it's totally different and very unique, so you'll be able to set yourself aside from the competition. That means you can charge what you want, you create your own market.

Creating Value First, Set Fees Second

That's one of the brilliant things I learned at a conference with Tim Ferriss in Boulder, Colorado. Tim Ferriss sets himself apart from the competition because what he does cannot be duplicated. He doesn't choose to go into a venture and compete for the lowest price; he prefers to offer his content as free or for a very high dollar amount event. I see too many recent graduates of acupuncture school fret needlessly over how much to charge for their services. If that is the concern in your mind, you are asking the wrong question. The best use of your energy would be to ask, "How can I offer enough of a transformative experience in my treatments that people would value it to the point of paying me higher than the average fee?" Then the next question is, "How can I best bundle my services and treatments around the goal of getting the result (back pain resolved, hormones regulated, autoimmune corrected, etc.) that this patient came in for?" In my book, *Healthcare on Purpose*, you can learn more about this concept.

If you're a community acupuncture clinic and you set up next to another community acupuncture clinic, then what you're selling is a commodity because you're just battling with prices. I am sure the experience of working with you is amazing, but many acupuncturists lose sight of the truth that people will pay for what they value. By lowering fees, you decrease the value people see that you provide in many cases. You think that your practice is slow because you charge too much or because of the economy, so you lower your fees and then end up out of business, and I've seen it hundreds of times. What structural alignment acupuncture does is it gives you a blank canvas where you can paint in your own art and your art is worth whatever you name it to be.

Bundle Your Fees and Services

You'll help enough people in an impactful way that helps them feel incredibly good and they have more confidence in you because of your connection with them and your needling skills; they're willing to do whatever you recommend. If you say, "Look, I want to get you on a wellness program," they say, "Great, sign me up." You'll say, "Okay, that's going to be this test. There's going to be coaching, there's going to be classes.

I'm going to take you through A to Z and we're going to recover your health," and they'll say, "Sign me up. I love what you've done for me so far and I want to be part of your wellness program and I'm happy to invest $5,000 in my health for your program."

Maybe their investment is more or less but that's not the going to hold them back because they already know that it will be money well spent based on how much value you have offered them.

When you can create confidence and certainty, then you can start using the other tools that you've learned in Chinese medicine, which some of that could be herbal medicine. It might be nutrition, (hopefully you learned some great nutrition). Qigong will be another service. You can offer meditation and mindfulness, that's all part of the medicine. Then you can start branching out and you can really start offering what truly is Chinese medicine. This will give you that bridge. It's a funnel, it's a conduit. When you bundle all of your acupuncture and the rest of the five branches of Chinese medicine into a comprehensive program, then you can actually get lasting results. People want the final solution and they know that their lifestyle has to be addressed, they understand that data needs to be collected from labs, and now more than ever, they want help reducing their stress levels.

Sotai Ho Exercises and Flow

Back to Sotai Ho. Take a minute, stand up and just march in place. Now bring your left knee up and your right knee and see which one comes up higher.

Okay, so if you are testing and your left knee comes up higher, then march in place about 15 times and you're just barely going to bring your right knee up, just a little bit, but your left knee, you're going to over-exaggerate it, because remember, we're moving in the path that your body likes to go. You're going to over-exaggerate it about 15 times and then recheck by marching to see if both knees feel like they're coming up equally. The cool thing about that is, as they come up equally, then you're realigning your spine, so once again, you have better digestion, you're going to have fewer issues with knee pain and ankle pain and degeneration, all from that simple exercise, and your patients will love that.

The other exercise you can do is you can lie on your back and you can bend your knees at a 45-degree angle, drop them to the left, and drop them to the right. Which side do you like going to the most? Whatever side you like going to the most, then you're going to stretch to that side. All these movements that Dr. Hashimoto combined, he actually found a way to decrease pain.

Most of my patients, I can get them out of 80% of pain just with Sotai Ho.

It's brilliant because, for those patients who are afraid of needles, there's no problem. Just do some Sotai Ho movement therapy. Once you master Sotai Ho, then you can really start to understand how the structure of the body works. Once you understand the physical structure, which is your foundation, then you start to understand the physiology behind the structure. When you have a structural distortion that's affecting the physiology, and once you understand that, then you say, "Wow, well, how is that physiology affecting the chemistry? And how's that chemistry affecting the neurochemistry? And how's the bacterial environment affecting the hormones?" It all weaves together.

This is a very powerful method that is going to transform your practice and transform your life. The next patient you find, I want you to do that simple marching exercise in place. Have them bring their right leg up and their left and see which one feels the best, and then take a note of that. Look at their spine and if their left knee comes up higher than their right, in most cases, 90% of cases, what you'll find is you go to do their lower back diagnostics, you'll find that, sure enough, their left hip is higher than their right. It became easier for them to lift their left leg up and it was creating a little bit of an imbalance.

Over time, that left-hip contraction is what's going to cause a lot of issues, like constipation, which can lead to leaky gut, it can lead to Dysbiosis, to a yeast overgrowth, and it can lead to ulcerative colitis. It can lead to so many different things, so with your ability to diagnose these patterns of disharmony and patterns of distortion, you'll have a much easier chance of getting rid and preventing these chronic diseases that are so prevalent in our society today.

Leading Causes of Death

In October of 2016, The Centers for Disease Control released the number of deaths for leading causes of death report which are:

- Heart disease: 614,348
- Cancer: 591,699
- Chronic lower respiratory diseases: 147,101
- Accidents (unintentional injuries): 136,053
- Stroke (cerebrovascular diseases): 133,103
- Alzheimer's disease: 93,541
- Diabetes: 76,488
- Influenza and Pneumonia: 55,227
- Nephritis, nephrotic syndrome and nephrosis: 48,146
- Intentional self-harm (suicide): 42,773

We've got to do more to prevent these diseases from happening. It's almost depressing to think that heart disease is still the leading cause of death today. Speaking of depression—if you are depressed by the health of America, then I will write you out a Prozac script. No, I'm joking. Nobody's Prozac deficient anyway, but what you'll find on the CDC is 75% of patient visits to doctors is pharmaceutical-based. We've got to change that.

We need doctors' visits to be herb-based and acupuncture-based and something lifestyle-based. My challenge to you is to create bridges in your community with medical doctors. You will find that we are all on the same team, we just play different positions.

Action Item: Make a list of five clinics that you will stop by and introduce yourself in the next seven days.

Repeat this process every week.

Rooted in the Foundational Acupuncture Points

Welcome to Chapter 4 in *Acupuncture Blueprint for Success*. I'm so happy you made it this far. Hopefully, you're taking notes and trying these things out. This is a very hands-on approach to care, so get on our website and sign up for an upcoming event and meet some of the coolest acupuncturists on the planet! But before the event I want you to be saying, "Prove it to me, Regan. Does this really work?" The only way I can prove it to you is if actually try it and watch your results increase. All I know is that you have to first commit yourself 100% to trying things differently, then grow a pair and start doing it. The results come later.

The Functions of the Points

What are the functions of the kidneys? Think about how powerful they are in balancing electrolytes and fluids. They also allow us to take a nice deep inhalation. Emotionally, too much fear can disturb our kidneys, our water element, but the kidney is also where we cultivate wisdom. From the old Chinese saying, that's where the big dipper pours out its destiny into our kidneys and then our kidneys hold our life's purpose.

The beautiful thing is the kidneys also house our Jing. Similar to your telomere length on your DNA. How long's your telomere? Have you had yours tested yet?

How do you locate the Kidney shu? You draw a line from the lower rib cage, you bring it across, or you can go three intervertebral spaces up from large intestine shu. Needle that point, use about an inch and a half needle, go in about an inch. Wait for that sweet spot, that gumminess and wait for the body to say, "Yeah, I've had enough, that's where it needs to go." As you listen to the body, the body will tell you that's the right depth and you go the right depth, and then you go to the next kidney point and do the same.

Then you go up to the spleen shu. The spleen shu, once again that's going to be about three intervertebral spaces up. You're going to needle the spleen shu, the same principle. Spleen shu is for people who have fibromyalgia, chronic fatigue, people who don't digest their food well, lots of undigested food in their stool. They have symptoms of hypothyroidism, they may be losing their hair, and they may be anemic. They may even have blood sugar issues. You're going to be feeling for that induration, that little sesame seed in this point and you're not going to find it, it's going to spit your needle out.

You're going to have to go in there and get a little aggressive with your diabetic patients or patients who are American and crave sweets. Put the needle in, get a tugging response, and pull it out. Go up to the liver shu, this is two cun up from that, two intervertebral spaces. The most accurate way to find the Liver shu is to take a surgical pen and draw a horizontal line connecting the lower border of the scapula. Take a step back and determine which side is lower, then you can see which side of the upper back is most contracted. Is their right shoulder pulled down, or is their left? This becomes your secondary weight bias.

Once you get a diagnostic pattern, then you'll see that the side that's contracted which allows you to understand where you are going to needle a little deeper. You may also needle about three or four extra points on the contracted side based on where you find indurations.

The first point to needle on the contracted side is the liver shu. The Liver shu is going to be great for your patients who are irritable, the patients who get headaches, patients who are inflexible, patients who are grumpy in the morning and look like they swallowed a bowling ball. They can be jerks, they can make everyone feel stressed when they come in the office. Have you noticed when, all of a sudden, the team scatters like cockroaches when certain patients come in?

These are your liver patients. These are also patients who have maybe acne or painful menses.

When the liver point is reactive, you're going to want to make sure that first of all, you're testing their hormones. Second, you're getting them in some type of stretching routine, take them through some Sotai-Hō movements. Third, you're going to get them on the right herbs. Chai Hu is one of the best things you can give them. You can inject Chai Hu into that liver shu point if that's legal in your state. Finally, test their MTHFR and entire methylation cycle to determine if they are converting methionine into glutathione. If not, they will end up with elevated homocysteine. If they do in fact have a mutation in this genetic pathway, then you will need to support this pathway. Otherwise, their liver will become inflamed and this will impede your ability to realign their spine with acupuncture.

Now we go to the diaphragm shu. Diaphragm shu is going to help the people who have any issues with their blood—any hemophiliacs, don't treat them. Anyone who has amenorrhea, dysmenorrhea, chronic fatigue or fibromyalgia. Anyone who's got issues with maybe Lyme disease, anyone who has Epstein-Barr virus, cytomegalovirus or hepatitis.

The diaphragm shu influences the blood and impacts the adult stem cell proliferation in regards to auto-immune issues in the blood. You're going to needle into the diaphragm shu very carefully because what's under your needle? Think about the risks. The lungs, right? Don't needle these points deep until you learn how; you will need hands-on training to needle the upper back points properly. I'm not even going to explain the needling technique beyond just find the induration, put the needle in and move on, but put the needle in perpendicular, don't do the oblique stuff. That actually is more dangerous in my opinion, unless you're going shallow on the needle but then you miss the induration, so all these points are perpendicular.

You needle the diaphragm shu, once again you're going to find the induration and needle this point bilaterally. Go ahead and needle the contracted side first and then move up to the next point. What is the next point? The next point is one cun up is your governing vessel shu. This is the point that is one of the most important points you're going to needle because it will open up the energy pathways on the entire spine. The governing vessel runs along the midline of the body and manifests along the spine. This meridian connects the kidneys to the heart to the brain and is one of the most essential meridian systems for spirituality. This is considered the cosmic loop from a Zen Buddhist perspective.

When you needle the GV points, you open energy cycles along their spine and down into their organs.

Now you're moving up to the heart point. This point is one of the most powerful points as well because this is where a person can really open up and start to feel authentic. I find in treating the heart shu that patients get emotional or they may bring up certain feelings of gratitude and they relax and you get to experience just how cool your patients are and how many unique individuals there are. Even though there are seven billion humans, I love all humans. I think there are so many cool stories and so many cool people.

As you needle their heart shu, that's when you're allowing them to express who they are as a person, as an individual. I think it can be a very beautiful process. You needle those points and that person starts to wake up. Their timing is better. They actually start to joke, you can feel some joy coming through. That's because you needle it just right and your finger pressure has to be right. You're not going to be slamming them on the table like some big old Russian bodybuilder who got banned from the Olympics. You're going to be nice and gentle.

As you're palpating these points, as you're needling these points, you're going to be very patient as you put the needles in. This is not a rushed process, but once you get proficient at this treatment, it really only takes about six to seven minutes. I've timed myself on tens of thousands of treatments and seven minutes is about the average when you get really in your flow state and start doing this. Yes, you can help a lot of people and you can build a very successful practice where you're actually adding more value, more quality, because remember, people want your expertise a lot more than they want your time. When needling the heart point, they start to open up.

The next point you find, which is very powerful, it's the gao huang shu at bladder 44. This point is often referred to as the happy point because of the story of an emperor who was terminally ill and called on all of the most noteworthy physicians of the time and none of them were able to diagnose him. Finally, a physician from far away was able to listen to the pulse and determine that the emperor had a pathogen in the gao huang area—the space between the pericardium and the heart—and it would be terminal unless the pathogen was released. The physician needled Bladder 44 and released the pathogen and the emperor began recovering and everyone was happy; hence the name the happy point.

If you dig a little deep into this point and its functions, it does calm the shen and opens the heart and there are some studies around serotonin metabolites increasing after acupuncture on the gao huang shu. At East West Health, we test neurotransmitter metabolites through urine. It's incredible how much better people feel when they balance their neurotransmitters. Serotonin, in general, gets increased with acupuncture, but this point has a more profound effect on the neurotransmitters. If you're not doing neurotransmitter testing, I highly recommend you start getting it in your practice because it can add a huge value when you balance a person's dopamine, their serotonin, their anandamide, and GABA, they start feeling more connected and alive. There are many things you can do for them that are non-drug based.

When you properly needle the gao huang shu, the person starts to feel this nice release. Then you go to San Jiao 15, this is where a lot of people hold their stress and they will love you forever when you release this point. You can also choose Gallbladder 21 or San Jiao 15, or both based on indurations and structural misalignment. The upper trapezius is where so many of us hold our tension, especially those of you who are on a computer all day, you get needled in that point all of a sudden you're like, "Wow, thank you," because you will feel a sense of relief.

You'll probably feel the muscle contract initially and then the whole thing will relax because remember when the needle hits those spindle cells the whole muscle gets retrained. Instead of being contracted, you're changing that nerve response so the muscle can relax and that person can actually get a better range of motion. They'll start feeling more alive, they'll start feeling more at peace—acupuncture, the solution for world peace.

Give these points a try and I think you're going to notice that your patients are going to be so happy. They're going to get off the table and they're going to smile and you will see the sincere gratitude on their face.

Then the final points you're going to look at are going to be gallbladder 20. You're going to go back and palpate, find the mastoid process, let your finger slide into that groove and then slip the needle into gallbladder 20, which will help their immune system, help with headaches, help their eyesight. Don't force this needle in, let it slide in very gently. Otherwise, you will cause discomfort; you could give them a hematoma and they will suddenly start questioning your skills. Acupuncture is amazing when done properly, and my goal is to help you find your authentic self in the process.

Structural Alignment Acupuncture may seem simple, but the results are profound for you and your patients.

Receiving Acupuncture for Your Own Experience and Rejuvenation

Of all the great services we provide in our clinics at East West Health, acupuncture is still the coolest. I know many of you have been to my clinic and you've seen it. Maybe some of you have actually received treatments there, but the acupuncture is amazing. I've had stem cell therapy, I've done all the IVs, run multiple functional medicine labs, herbal injections, but acupuncture is still, in my heart of hearts, the most beautiful medicine available.

My challenge to you is to go find an acupuncturist. Get out there and get networking. Find an acupuncturist and get treated. If you have a good friend who can treat you, call them today. I know a lot of us are friends. Call me up. I'll give you a treatment, but it's going to cost you $8,000. No, I'm joking, I'd love to treat you. That's one of the things we do at our Structural Alignment Acupuncture workshops. We work on each other and we get everybody feeling real good, real loving, and real impactful.

Anchoring Points for Structural Alignment

The Acupuncture Anchors

Let's dive into the final insights of the Structural Alignment Acupuncture training. It's been such a fun process, but I'll see you again, stay connected. Once you've mastered needling the back shu points, you will feel a higher level of confidence. You'll see the way you can detect if your treatment worked is by the way your patient's face looks. You'll notice they look younger, they have fewer wrinkles. Maybe they've been lying face down. If they have water retention, they're going to have more wrinkles, but you're going to notice that their eyes just look happier, they look clearer, they look more pristine. They have a nice smile on their face. That's one of your biggest gauges. The next one is watching for the decrease of indurations and the improvement in their posture. They will become more upright and spiritual.

One of the key procedures is to needle the anchor points before you treat the spine. If you just do the Back Shu points only, there are a few points that you don't want to miss. Otherwise, that could blow the entire treatment. One of the points that you want to needle is large intestine 10. Large intestine 10 is right on the brachioradialis.

Sometimes you can even turn their palm of their hand, you can supinate it or pronate it, and you'll find that induration will pop out, then you'll needle right into that induration. Large intestinal 11 is also an option. You simply find the induration, and then needle that point if there's an induration there. That will help anchor all the upper back points.

If you don't use an anchor, then sometimes people get a headache after this treatment because it's a massive realignment. I know the first time I got chiropractic, I had a massive headache, and I was like, "Wow, never mind," because there's no anchoring in it. There was no massage, nothing to get my blood moving away from my head and my neck. I'd highly recommend, don't forget to do these points. This is part of the overall structural alignment protocol. You can use a point like San Jiao 5 or San Jiao 6, those can also be anchoring points that you can use.

Do some type of anchoring point; the traditional points are large intestine 10, large intestine 11. Then, you go down to the legs. Let's talk about large intestine 10, large intestine 11 just for a minute because I think if you visualize what they do to your physiology you will appreciate them more. They help with the connective tissue, they relax the fascia, and they also are great points for building up immunity.

Of course, if you've got viral infection, a sore throat, any kind of heat in the body, large intestine 11 is going to be beautiful. Most Americans need that point because of chronic inflammation. That's the killer in our country: the inflammatory diseases like cancer, heart disease, and diabetes. What you'll do is you'll want to make sure that you're looking and visualizing what effect these points are going to have on the digestive system as well as the musculoskeletal system.

Once you've done those points, then you're going to drop down at the legs. You're going to palpate stomach 36. Once again, this is going to be more distal than the Chinese. This is going to be about two cun below the tibial tuberosity. You're going to needle into that point right against the tibia, this is one of the best points for building white blood cells in the body. It helps with gastric secretions, improves digestion. As you know, this is one of the major points for endurance. A lot of my athletes, they love this point. They feel great when they get it. It's also good for your patients who are immunocompromised.

You'll also want to palpate Gallbladder 34. Gallbladder 34 is actually more proximal than the TCM location. You're going to want to go to find Gallbladder 34, go up about a half cun and that's the typical location for structural alignment.

This point helps relax the iliotibial band. It's great for headaches. It's great for detoxification if you're working on your liver patients. It also helps patients just fall into deeper states of relaxation, They'll recover quicker from their runs. Needle those points, that's the finishing.

In Seitai Shinpo, we'd use moxibustion. In the Structural Alignment Acupuncture method, we send them home with more herbs, more nutrition, and more lifestyle guidance. That's one of the big differences here. But feel free to moxa, if you know how to do direct moxa, put some cones on these points, it can help a lot. You want to palpate and sense how their organs are, do a hara diagnosis. Just feel the person's belly. Patients feel so connected to you when you come into the room, you just take a minute to connect and tell them what's going on with their body in the present moment. I find using pulse and tongue diagnostics are very simple, they don't take a lot of time if you are good at them.

The most important process is learning how to connect with your patients. You do a hara diagnosis, "Yeah, something feels wrong with your intestines, we need to do a stool profile." They say "Yeah, absolutely, that was so painful when you pushed on that point." The more you connect with your patients through bringing high levels of energy, intention, and skill, the happier you will be as a practitioner.

The methods you've learned will only work when you are a clear conduit and 100% receptive to the patterns showing up in front of you.

Creating a Transformative, Fun, and Bigger Future

I've just got to say how honored I am that you made it this far. You've tried new things. You're opening up your mind to a whole new world of acupuncture. I've taken you through the majority of the acupuncture points in the structural alignment method. The only thing we haven't touched on are the limbs, the peripheral—the branches, so to speak. We're going to touch on that right now, but I just have to thank each one of you for who you are. The amount of work that you put into your career, your profession, the amount of people who have gone before us, my hat's off to you.

I've sat on the Utah Acupuncture licensing board for about five years now. I have to say, it's not an easy process but I can't give enough thanks to those who have set the foundation before me for what they've done with the legislature, getting things known to the public. I think we've just scratched the surface with the influence we can make. For those of you who are taking my courses, I know you've got a bigger purpose, you've got a bigger vision, you're willing to invest in your training, invest in your health, invest in learning something new. I find that's one of the most distinguishable characteristics of a successful acupuncturist. It's somebody who digs in and commits to learn.

Some of you may go crazy when I say this, but I spend almost six figures a year on training courses, on learning, on my mentors, on mastering the medicine, learning new things, bringing in new programs. I find that's the best money spent. The return that I get on the training and coaching that I receive is at least 10 to 1 because I implement and make the changes. I really believe that I can have an impact on changing the way healthcare is delivered in America and especially in your practice. My genius is in helping healthcare practitioners become entrepreneurs. I help practitioners just like you find their bigger future and transformative purpose because that's what's needed to get us out of the current pattern the world is in now.

I can't wait to meet those of you who want to make a bigger impact and have a bigger future. I look forward to becoming friends with you and learning from you. Get out to one of our events. We've got our healthcare entrepreneur program. We take you through four sessions in our healthcare entrepreneur program so that you become a black belt in running a successful clinic. The first training helps your find your voice and art and is called, "*Leaning on Kanye West to Transform Healthcare in America*", or **Session 1**. "*Thinking like Elon Musk to Disrupt Healthcare in America*" is **Session 2**.

I've created "*Einstein's Equation for Creating an Amazing Medicine of the Future*" is **Session 3**, and **Session 4** is "*The Tao of the Healthcare Entrepreneur*." These trainings will move your future in a much more engaging way when it comes to thinking about growing your office as the leader of a Dojo. Many of my clients are now running seven-figure clinics and are helping more people than they ever imagined.

I've also created the 4-Level Functional Medicine Boot Camps. For the **Acupuncture Blueprint for Success** program, we train on Structural Alignment Acupuncture, which I want to see all of you at. If you like what you've read and learned so far, then reach out to me. I'd love to meet you. One of life's greatest gifts is in meeting like-minded individuals. They feel like family to me. I may give you a big hug, so watch out!

Here's to a bigger future than you ever imagined!

All the best,

Regan Archibald, Lac, CSSAc
Functional Medicine Practitioner

Here's How to Transform Your Practice Growth and Clinical Results 10x with Structural Alignment Acupuncture

You already know that acupuncture yields incredible results and reverses some of the toughest conditions. The struggle that we're all faced with is how do we master the medicine and grow a vibrant, thriving acupuncture practice at the same time?

That's where we come in. We help acupuncturists just like you grow your acupuncture practice so you can help more people than you've ever dreamed of.

Step 1: We give you the training modules that you need that give you expert business systems so that you can help people in a stress-free way.

Step 2: We provide is incredible mentorship on a one-of-a-kind acupuncture art called structural alignment acupuncture so that you can correct spinal distortions and reverse autoimmune conditions.

Step 3: You get is a step by step approach to effectively deliver a report of findings that will double or triple your revenue.

Most acupuncturists spend years mastering the art of acupuncture and the craft of their skill, but never learn how to help a lot of people because they don't take the time to learn how to run a business.

Now you can grow your acupuncture practice and help more people than you ever dreamed of. If you'd like us to help, just email us at: **Info@GoWellness.com** and we'll take it from there.

About Me

Regan's curiosity about health started at an early age. In his teens, he began researching how to improve human performance, memory, and strength. His keen interest in health and well-being led him to the University of Utah where he prepared for medical school. During his undergraduate studies, he came to the conclusion that the allopathic medical approach of using drugs and surgery for patients was not the way he wanted to help people.

He realized that his true passion was in holistic medicine and set off for training in Hawaii. Regan graduated with his Masters of Science from the Traditional Chinese Medical College of Hawaii and went on to found East West Health in 2004.

East West Health is one of the few clinics in the nation to successfully integrate traditional eastern medicine and functional western medicine. Throughout his career, Regan has been a prolific writer, speaker, teacher and instructor. He is the author of *Your Health Transformation* and *Healthcare on Purpose* and has created over 15 educational courses to enlighten and inspire patients and healthcare providers.

Regan shares his knowledge on his popular health podcast called *Go Wellness Radio*. He has also produced training programs for healthcare providers to enhance their patient results and skill levels through **Go Wellness.com**. His purpose is to help individuals find freedom and independence when it comes to their health.